PARKINSON'S DISEASE DIET COOKBOOK

Essential Recipes For Managing Symptoms, Boosting Brain Health, And Enhancing Mobility With Nutrient-Rich, Anti-Inflammatory Meals

DR ELIAN GRIFFIN

DISCLAIMER

The nutritional recommendations and recipes in this book are meant solely for informative reasons. They are not meant to replace the counsel, diagnosis, or care of a qualified medical expert. If you have any doubts about a medical condition or dietary requirements, you should always see your physician or another trained healthcare expert.

All reasonable efforts have been taken by the author and publisher to ensure that the information contained in this book is correct as of the date of publication. Recommendations may alter, though, as medical knowledge is always changing. When using any of the recipes or instructions found here, the user assumes all liability and assumes no risk, whether personal or otherwise. People who have certain dietary requirements or medical issues should speak with a healthcare provider for personalized guidance. The given recipes are only ideas; you may need to adjust them to suit your own nutritional needs, tastes, and tolerances.

When you use this book, you agree to release the publisher, the author, and their representatives from any liability for any claims, damages, liabilities, costs, or expenditures resulting from your use of the book.

TABLE OF CONTENTS

CHAPTER ONE 13

  PARKINSON'S DISEASE DIET INTRODUCTION 13

    DIET IS CRUCIAL FOR MANAGING PARKINSON'S DISEASE 13

    AN OVERVIEW OF THE EFFECTS OF DIET ON SYMPTOMS..................14

    A SPECIALIZED COOKBOOK'S BENEFITS FOR PARKINSON'S 16

    THE WAY THIS BOOK IS ORGANIZED TO ASSIST YOU 18

    USING THE COOKBOOK WISELY TO RAISE LIVING STANDARDS 20

CHAPTER TWO 23

  COMPREHENDING PARKINSON'S DISEASE 23

    KNOWING THE SYMPTOMS OF PARKINSON'S DISEASE 23

    HOW NUTRITION IS ESSENTIAL FOR MANAGING SYMPTOMS...........24

    COMMON DIETARY OBSTACLES FOR PARKINSON'S PATIENTS 25

    NUTRITION'S ROLE IN OVERALL HEALTH...26

    A SYNOPSIS OF THE MOST RECENT DIETARY GUIDELINES 27

CHAPTER THREE 29

  CREATING THE BASIS OF YOUR PARKINSON'S DIET 29

    KEYS TO A PARKINSON'S DISEASE-FRIENDLY DIET 29

    FOODS TO CONSUME TO MANAGE SYMPTOMS................................30

    FOODS TO REFRAIN FROM OR REDUCE 32

    THE EFFECTS OF HYDRATION AND THEIR IMPORTANCE...................33

    SAMPLE MENUS FOR VARIOUS PARKINSON'S DISEASE STAGES 34

CHAPTER FOUR 37

  ESSENTIAL DIETS FOR PEOPLE WITH PARKINSON'S DISEASE 37

    IMPORTANT ELEMENTS THAT ARE GOOD FOR PARKINSON'S
    PATIENTS 37

THE USE OF SUPPLEMENTS TO HELP WITH SYMPTOM 38

TECHNIQUES FOR COOKING THAT MAINTAIN NUTRIENTS 39

RECIPES PACKED WITH VITAL MINERALS AND VITAMINS 40

INCLUDING PROTEIN FOR HEALTHY MUSCLES AND ENERGY 41

CHAPTER FIVE 43

COOKING METHODS AND ADVICE 43

SIMPLE COOKING METHODS FOR PARKINSON'S DISEASE PATIENTS .43

EQUIPMENT & TOOLS FOR PREPARING MEALS 44

MAKING MEALS AHEAD OF TIME FOR CONVENIENCE 45

HOW TO ADJUST RECIPES TO FIT SPECIFIC DIETARY REQUIREMENTS
....46

STRATEGIES FOR HANDLING TIREDNESS WHEN COOKING 47

CHAPTER SIX 49

PARTICULAR DAYS AND FESTIVITIES 49

ORGANIZING LUNCHES FOR PARTICULAR EVENTS...........................49

RECIPES FOR FAMILY GET-TOGETHERS 50

ADAPTING CLASSIC RECIPES TO MEET DIETARY REQUIREMENTS......51

IDEAS FOR ENJOYING THE HOLIDAYS WITH FRIENDS AND FAMILY ...52

STRATEGIES FOR HANDLING DIETARY LIMITATIONS DURING
HOLIDAYS 53

CHAPTER SEVEN 55

MEAL PLANNING: BREAKFASTS RECIPES 55

HEALTHY BREAKFAST CHOICES TO BEGIN THE DAY 55

SIMPLE AND FAST BREAKFAST RECIPES 56

WORTH OF A WELL-BALANCED BREAKFAST......................................57

RECIPES FOR INCREASED VITALITY 58

BREAKFAST CONCEPTS FIT FOR A RANGE OF DIETARY 59

PARKINSON'S DISEASE PATIENTS' LUNCHES AND DINNERS...................61

CHOOSING HEALTHFUL LUNCH AND DINNER OPTIONS.....................61

ONE-POT DINNERS FOR EASE...62

DINNER RECIPES THAT ARE FAMILY-FRIENDLY 63

IDEAS FOR EASY LUNCHES..65

HEALTHY MEALS TO CONTROL SYMPTOMS ALL DAY LONG...............66

DESSERTS & SNACKS FOR A PARKINSON'S DIET.......................................68

HEALTHY SNACK IDEAS TO REDUCE CRAVINGS..................................68

DESSERTS THAT ARE HEALTHFUL BUT NOT GUILTY 69

THE VALUE OF PORTION MANAGEMENT IN SNACKS.........................70

RECIPES FOR DESSERTS AND SNACKS MADE AT HOME 71

LIMITING SUGAR CONSUMPTION WHILE INDULGING IN SWEETS.....72

SMOOTHIES AND BEVERAGES FOR PARKINSON'S DISEASE 74

DRINKS THAT ARE HYDRATING FOR PEOPLE WITH PARKINSON'S 74

NUTRIENT-PACKED SMOOTHIE RECIPES 75

THE VALUE OF MAINTAINING HYDRATION DURING THE DAY 76

SUGGESTIONS FOR WARM AND CHILLED DRINKS 77

DRINKS TO LIMIT OR STEER CLEAR OFF TO MANAGE SYMPTOMS 78

CHAPTER EIGHT...81

FAQS AND LIFESTYLE ADVICE 81

THE BENEFITS OF EXERCISE FOR MANAGING PARKINSON'S
SYMPTOMS 81

SLEEP IS ESSENTIAL FOR GENERAL HEALTH 82

CONTROLLING STRESS AND HOW IT AFFECTS SYMPTOMS...............83

COMMON QUESTIONS REGARDING PARKINSON'S DISEASE AND......84

SOURCES OF ADDITIONAL INFORMATION AND SUPPORT.................85

ABOUT THE BOOK

The "Parkinson's Disease Diet Cookbook" is an invaluable tool for anyone navigating the challenges of controlling Parkinson's disease through dietary interventions. Readers who live with this condition must comprehend the significant influence of diet on symptom management. The cookbook equips readers with the necessary knowledge to make educated dietary decisions by giving a thorough overview of Parkinson's disease and its symptoms.

With detailed meal plans tailored to different stages of the disease, readers can easily adapt their diets to suit their changing needs. This specialized cookbook addresses common challenges faced by patients with Parkinson's disease and offers practical strategies to overcome them through nutrition. It outlines the principles of a Parkinson's-friendly diet, highlighting foods that aid in symptom management while emphasizing the importance of hydration and balanced nutrition.

Nutritional necessities are covered in detail, with an emphasis on important nutrients and supplements that help manage symptoms. The cookbook encourages cooking methods that maintain these necessities so that meals are not only nourishing but also fun to make. Recipes high in protein, which are critical for keeping muscles healthy and energy levels high, are highlighted in particular.

Specifically designed for Parkinson's patients, these useful cooking tips and techniques provide simple, straightforward instructions and suggest adaptive tools to make meal preparation easier.

They also cover strategies for coping with cooking fatigue, which adds to the practicality and lessens the stress that comes with mealtimes.

For holidays and special events, the cookbook offers meal-planning advice and holiday-appropriate recipes so that Parkinson's patients can partake in celebratory meals without sacrificing their dietary requirements. It also promotes modifying classic recipes to meet particular health needs, which promotes inclusivity at social events.

The cookbook highlights the significance of snacks and desserts that are both healthy and satisfying, encouraging portion control and mindful eating habits. It offers a wide array of meal ideas designed to support symptom management throughout the day, from wholesome breakfast options to balanced lunch and dinner recipes.

The importance of hydration and providing creative drink ideas that accommodate a variety of tastes and dietary restrictions are highlighted in this cookbook, along with nutrient-dense smoothie recipes and drink options that are ideal for managing symptoms and preserving general health.

Beyond nutrition, the cookbook covers lifestyle aspects that are critical to treating Parkinson's disease, such as the need for exercise, sleep, and stress reduction.

Frequently asked issues are thoroughly addressed, offering clarification and further resources for continuing assistance and knowledge.

The "Parkinson's Disease Diet Cookbook" is essentially a comprehensive guide designed to improve the quality of life for individuals with Parkinson's disease by incorporating informed food decisions and lifestyle modifications, rather than merely a compilation of recipes.

CHAPTER ONE

DIET IS CRUCIAL FOR MANAGING PARKINSON'S DISEASE

Maintaining a well-balanced diet that is customized to support overall health and effectively manage symptoms is an important part of managing Parkinson's disease. Dietary factors influence neurotransmitter function and reduce inflammation, which in turn influences the management of symptoms like tremors, rigidity, and bradykinesia. Antioxidant, vitamin, and mineral-rich diets protect neurons and support brain health. Proper nutrition also improves medication effectiveness and minimizes side effects, which promotes better symptom management and overall well-being.

Dietary factors that affect Parkinson's disease symptoms are important to understand because certain foods and nutrients can either exacerbate or alleviate symptoms. For example, the timing of protein intake can affect the absorption of levodopa, a key medication for

Parkinson's, while foods high in antioxidants, such as fruits and vegetables, can have neuroprotective effects. People can better manage fluctuations in their symptoms and improve their quality of life by adopting a diet that balances protein intake with other nutrients.

A well-planned, nutrient-dense diet can have a substantial impact on the course and treatment of Parkinson's disease. A diet rich in whole foods, lean proteins, healthy fats, and an abundance of fruits and vegetables can promote general health, reduce drug interactions, and increase energy levels. Additionally, keeping a healthy weight can lessen the strain on joints and muscles, which can lead to increased mobility and functional ability. Individuals with Parkinson's disease who place a high priority on nutrition can empower themselves to better manage their condition and maximize their quality of life overall.

AN OVERVIEW OF THE EFFECTS OF DIET ON SYMPTOMS

Nutrition is a key factor in controlling the symptoms of Parkinson's disease because it affects neurotransmitter levels and maintains brain health in general. Some nutrients, like the omega-3 fatty acids in fish and flaxseed, can help reduce inflammation and support neuronal health. On the other hand, too much protein can interfere with the absorption of levodopa, which can affect the effectiveness of medication and exacerbate motor fluctuations. Vitamin B6, B12, and folate deficiencies can lead to cognitive decline and fatigue.

Adopting a diet that supports brain health and overall well-being can potentially slow down the progression of Parkinson's disease, enhance medication efficaciousness, and improve daily functioning. Eating a diet high in antioxidants, such as berries, leafy greens, and nuts, can help combat oxidative stress and protect neurons from damage. Staying hydrated is also important to prevent dehydration, which can worsen symptoms like constipation and cognitive impairment. Speaking with a registered dietitian can offer personalized guidance on nutrition strategies catered to individual needs and symptoms.

For those who have Parkinson's disease, a balanced diet can help reduce symptoms and enhance quality of life. It's important to stay away from processed foods that are high in sugar and unhealthy fats because these can worsen symptoms and cause inflammation. Instead, whole grains, lean proteins, and foods high in vitamins and minerals can support optimal brain function and provide sustained energy. People with Parkinson's disease can take charge of their health and maximize their well-being by learning how diet affects their symptoms and making educated dietary decisions.

A SPECIALIZED COOKBOOK'S BENEFITS FOR PARKINSON'S PATIENTS

Cookbooks with recipes that highlight nutrient-rich foods that are known to support brain health, such as fruits, vegetables, whole grains, and lean proteins, are a great way for patients with Parkinson's disease to manage their symptoms and maintain overall health. By following recipes that are specifically tailored to meet the nutritional needs of people with Parkinson's disease, patients can make meal planning easier and make sure they're getting the right balance of nutrients to support their condition.

Additionally, specialty cookbooks frequently offer advice and techniques for handling dietary obstacles that Parkinson's patients frequently encounter, such as the need for softer textures or difficulty swallowing. This helpful advice enables people with Parkinson's disease and those who care for them to modify recipes to suit particular dietary requirements and preferences while maintaining a fun and healthy meal experience. Furthermore, these cookbooks may offer insights into how particular ingredients or cooking techniques may affect the effectiveness of medication, enabling patients to maximize their treatment outcomes through informed dietary choices.

Beyond utility, Parkinson's patient cookbooks help create a sense of support and community by disseminating personal accounts, dietary advice, and cooking techniques from other people with the disease.

This can lessen feelings of loneliness and encourage people to actively manage their health through nutrition. Specialized cookbooks also help people with Parkinson's disease and their caregivers live better lives by encouraging a positive relationship with food and offering easily accessible recipes that balance health and taste.

THE WAY THIS BOOK IS ORGANIZED TO ASSIST YOU

With sections focusing on various aspects of meal planning and preparation, ranging from breakfast ideas to dinner recipes and snacks, this Parkinson's Disease Diet Cookbook offers comprehensive support for anyone looking to manage their condition through nutrition. It starts with an introduction to the role of diet in managing Parkinson's disease, highlighting key nutrients and dietary strategies to optimize health and symptom control.

Many different, simple-to-follow recipes in each section are made with well-known ingredients to be healthful and appropriate for people with Parkinson's disease.

The recipes are organized according to their nutritional value, so it's easy for people to find meals that suit their particular dietary requirements and preferences. The cookbook also offers helpful advice on how to improve medication absorption and reduce symptom fluctuations by changing ingredients, controlling portion sizes, and timing meals.

In addition to recipes, this cookbook contains educational materials about nutrition and Parkinson's disease, giving readers the ability to make knowledgeable dietary decisions. It also covers common dietary difficulties that people with Parkinson's encounter, like swallowing difficulties or sensory changes, providing adaptive cooking methods and substitute ingredient options. The cookbook is organized in an approachable manner, providing users with helpful advice and encouraging material, enabling them to navigate their nutritional journey with confidence and effectively manage their Parkinson's symptoms.

By streamlining meal planning, optimizing nutrition, and assisting with symptom management, effectively utilizing this Parkinson's Disease Diet Cookbook can greatly enhance quality of life. To get started, read through the cookbook's introduction sections, which offer insights into the advantages of particular nutrients and dietary strategies for Parkinson's disease. These insights will help you make well-informed decisions when choosing recipes and organizing meals that promote your general health and well-being.

Consider meal prepping or batch cooking to save time and ensure you have nutritious meals readily available, especially on days when managing symptoms may require more rest or assistance. When using the cookbook, give priority to recipes that incorporate nutrient-rich ingredients known to benefit brain health, such as omega-3 fatty acids, antioxidants, and vitamins essential for neurological function.

Experiment with different recipes to discover flavors and textures that appeal to your palate while meeting your nutritional needs.

As you explore your culinary options with this cookbook, record in a food diary how various meals and ingredients impact your symptoms and general well-being. This will allow you to determine which foods trigger or alleviate symptoms, which will help you make more informed dietary decisions over time. Additionally, maintain contact with your healthcare team, which should include a registered dietitian, to address any dietary concerns or modifications based on your specific health requirements and treatment plan.

Through the effective use of this cookbook, you can take proactive measures to improve your nutrition, better manage your Parkinson's symptoms, and ultimately live a higher quality of life. Seize the chance to try new flavors, include nourishing ingredients.

CHAPTER TWO

COMPREHENDING PARKINSON'S DISEASE

KNOWING THE SYMPTOMS OF PARKINSON'S DISEASE

Parkinson's disease, or Parkinson's disease (PD), is a progressive neurological disorder that impairs movement. It arises from damage or death of nerve cells in the brain, specifically in the substantia nigra. These cells produce dopamine, a chemical messenger that is essential for smooth, coordinated muscle movement. Parkinson's disease progresses by lowering dopamine levels, which can cause tremors, stiffness, slow movement (called bradykinesia), and difficulty with balance, and coordination, among other non-motor symptoms.

Parkinson's disease is diagnosed by reviewing the patient's medical history, performing a neurological examination, and occasionally ordering imaging tests such as MRIs or CT scans. The disease's early symptoms can be mild and vary from person to person, making diagnosis difficult. As the disease progresses, the symptoms become more noticeable and can have a major impact on daily life.

HOW NUTRITION IS ESSENTIAL FOR MANAGING SYMPTOMS

A balanced diet high in nutrients, antioxidants, and fiber supports general health and may help alleviate some symptoms of Parkinson's disease. Certain nutrients, such as antioxidants (found in fruits and vegetables) and omega-3 fatty acids (found in fish), may have neuroprotective effects and help reduce inflammation in the brain. Diet plays a critical role in managing the symptoms and overall health of Parkinson's disease.

Parkinson's patients may have dietary difficulties, such as dysphagia (difficulty chewing and swallowing), which can have an impact on the amount of nutrition they consume. Parkinson's medication interactions with certain foods or nutrients can also cause changes in appetite or gastrointestinal problems, such as constipation, which can also have an impact on the amount of nutrition they consume.

COMMON DIETARY OBSTACLES FOR PARKINSON'S PATIENTS

Dysphagia, which can make chewing and swallowing difficult, is one common dietary challenge that Parkinson's patients often face. This can lead to reduced food intake, weight loss, and an increased risk of malnutrition. People with Parkinson's disease and their caregivers need to work with healthcare professionals, such as speech therapists or dietitians, to address these challenges and ensure adequate nutrition.

Finding the right balance between medication timing and meals is crucial for symptom management and general well-being. Managing medication and its interaction with food presents another challenge. For example, some Parkinson's medications, like levodopa, may need to be taken on an empty stomach to optimize absorption, while others may require food to minimize side effects like nausea.

Parkinson's patients may also have changes in taste and smell, which can impact appetite and food preferences; they may also have motor symptoms, such as tremors or stiffness, that make meal preparation and cooking difficult; however, adaptive strategies, like pre-cutting ingredients or using utensils with larger handles, can help make mealtime more enjoyable and manageable.

NUTRITION'S ROLE IN OVERALL HEALTH

A well-balanced diet supports immune function, bone health, and energy levels, all of which are critical for preserving quality of life. Adequate nutrition also helps manage common comorbidities associated with Parkinson's disease, such as cardiovascular disease and osteoporosis. Nutrition is an important aspect of overall health, particularly for individuals with Parkinson's disease.

Drinking plenty of water throughout the day is important for Parkinson's patients, as dehydration can worsen symptoms like fatigue and constipation. Nutrient-dense foods include fruits, vegetables, whole grains, lean proteins, and healthy fats. These foods also provide vital vitamins and minerals that support brain health and general well-being.

Another crucial component of managing Parkinson's disease is maintaining a healthy weight. While some people with the disease may gain weight unintentionally due to side effects from medications or reduced appetite, others may lose weight unintentionally due to decreased physical activity. Individuals with Parkinson's disease can benefit from working with a healthcare team to monitor nutritional status and make necessary dietary adjustments to maintain an optimal weight and improve overall health outcomes.

A SYNOPSIS OF THE MOST RECENT DIETARY GUIDELINES

A variety of nutrient-dense foods, such as fruits, vegetables, whole grains, lean proteins, and healthy fats, can provide essential vitamins and minerals that support brain health and energy levels. The current recommendations for diet for people with Parkinson's disease emphasize promoting a balanced and nutritious diet that supports overall health and symptom management.

To help manage weight and reduce inflammation, cutting back on processed foods, saturated fats, and added sugars may be beneficial for people with Parkinson's disease. Certain dietary patterns, like the Mediterranean diet, which is high in fruits, vegetables, whole grains, and healthy fats like olive oil and fish, may also have neuroprotective effects and improve the quality of life for people with Parkinson's disease.

A registered dietitian or other healthcare professional who specializes in Parkinson's disease can assist in developing a personalized nutrition plan that addresses specific dietary needs and goals. Regular monitoring and adjustments to the diet may be necessary as symptoms change or new challenges arise, ensuring optimal nutrition and overall well-being for people living with Parkinson's disease. Individualized nutrition plans may be necessary based on individual symptoms, medications, and personal preferences.

CHAPTER THREE

CREATING THE BASIS OF YOUR PARKINSON'S DIET

KEYS TO A PARKINSON'S DISEASE-FRIENDLY DIET

A Parkinson 's-friendly diet is based on principles that support overall health and effectively manage symptoms. The cornerstone of this approach is making sure that the diet is full of nutrients that support brain health and reduce inflammation, both of which are important in managing Parkinson's disease. Essential nutrients include whole foods like fruits, vegetables, whole grains, and lean proteins. These foods provide vital vitamins, minerals, and antioxidants that help combat oxidative stress, which is one of the factors that contributes to neurodegeneration in Parkinson's disease.

Additionally, focusing on foods that promote gut health, like probiotics found in yogurt and fermented foods, may help alleviate gastrointestinal issues commonly associated with Parkinson's disease. Portion control and regular meals throughout the day are also vital to stabilize energy levels and prevent fluctuations that can exacerbate symptoms. Finally, maintaining a balanced diet that includes adequate fiber helps support digestive health, which can be compromised in Parkinson's patients due to medication side effects.

In actuality, developing a Parkinson 's-friendly diet entails meal planning that integrates these ideas into regular eating routines. By giving nutrient-dense foods top priority and balancing macronutrients, people can optimize their diet to promote general well-being and effectively manage symptoms.

FOODS TO CONSUME TO MANAGE SYMPTOMS

Certain foods are essential for managing Parkinson's symptoms because they help reduce symptoms and support overall health. Antioxidant-rich foods like berries, spinach, and kale help fight inflammation and oxidative stress, two major factors that lead to neurodegeneration. Nuts and fatty fish like salmon contain omega-3 fatty acids, which support brain health and may help reduce symptoms like tremors and stiffness.

Including foods high in fiber, such as whole grains, fruits, and vegetables, supports digestive health and helps alleviate constipation, a common problem in Parkinson's disease. Maintaining adequate protein intake from lean sources like poultry, beans, and tofu supports muscle strength and overall energy levels. Vitamin D, obtained from sources like fortified dairy products and sunlight exposure, is important for bone health and may have protective effects on brain function.

A balanced approach including a variety of nutrient-rich foods guarantees comprehensive support for both physical and cognitive health. People can potentially improve their nutritional intake and alleviate some of the symptoms associated with Parkinson's disease by strategically incorporating these foods into daily meals and snacks.

Certain foods are recommended to be avoided or limited when managing Parkinson's disease because they may worsen symptoms or interfere with medication. High-fat and processed foods, such as fried foods and commercially baked goods, should be avoided because they can cause weight gain and inflammation, which can aggravate symptoms and overall health outcomes.

Coffee and alcohol should be consumed in moderation as they can interfere with medication effectiveness and exacerbate symptoms like tremors and insomnia. Excessive salt intake should also be avoided as it can lead to fluid retention and exacerbate blood pressure issues, which are common concerns in Parkinson's patients.

Furthermore, there may be a correlation between dairy consumption and an increased risk of Parkinson's progression, so people with Parkinson's disease should exercise caution when consuming dairy products.

By being aware of these dietary considerations and making educated decisions, people with Parkinson's disease can better manage their condition and promote overall well-being.

THE EFFECTS OF HYDRATION AND THEIR IMPORTANCE

Maintaining adequate hydration is essential for maintaining fluid balance, supporting kidney function, and facilitating medication absorption—all of which are critical for managing symptoms and optimizing treatment outcomes—especially for people with Parkinson's disease.

Dehydration can worsen symptoms like fatigue, constipation, and confusion, which are common in Parkinson's patients.

Drinking water regularly and eating foods high in water, like fruits and vegetables, help keep one's body hydrated. It's also worth noting that certain Parkinson's disease medications can raise the risk of dehydration, so it's even more critical to prioritize getting enough fluids.

By incorporating hydration as a fundamental aspect of daily self-care, people with Parkinson's disease can support their overall health and improve their quality of life.

Key strategies in maintaining optimal hydration include monitoring hydration status and adjusting fluid intake based on individual needs and environmental factors, such as temperature and activity level.

SAMPLE MENUS FOR VARIOUS PARKINSON'S DISEASE STAGES

In the early stages of the disease, concentrate on meals that include a variety of colorful fruits and vegetables, lean proteins like grilled chicken or fish, and whole grains like quinoa or brown rice. Including antioxidant-rich foods like berries and leafy greens that support brain health and fight oxidative stress.

These sample meal plans can help individuals manage their symptoms effectively while ensuring adequate nutrition and enjoyment of meals.

As Parkinson's disease worsens, meal plans should be modified to account for possible swallowing difficulties and decreased appetite.

You should choose softer textures and smaller, more frequent meals throughout the day to keep energy levels up and facilitate digestion. Healthy choices that are simpler to eat and digest include soups, smoothies, and pureed dishes.

In later stages, as swallowing and motor skills become more difficult, give preference to foods high in nutrients and easy to chew and swallow, like yogurt, oatmeal, and soft-cooked vegetables.

Eating meals that are well-balanced and contain enough protein, healthy fats, and complex carbohydrates promotes general health and aids in symptom management.

Individuals can optimize their nutritional intake, effectively manage their symptoms, and improve their quality of life by creating meal plans that are specifically tailored to their needs and stages of Parkinson's disease.

Speaking with a healthcare professional or nutritionist can offer personalized guidance and support in creating meal plans that are specific to dietary needs and preferences.

CHAPTER FOUR

ESSENTIAL DIETS FOR PEOPLE WITH PARKINSON'S DISEASE

IMPORTANT ELEMENTS THAT ARE GOOD FOR PARKINSON'S PATIENTS

For Parkinson's patients who may be at risk of bone thinning due to reduced mobility, a well-balanced diet that emphasizes nutrients that support brain health and overall well-being is essential. Antioxidants such as vitamins C and E, which help shield cells from damage caused by free radicals, omega-3 fatty acids, which are found in fish like salmon and flaxseeds, can reduce inflammation and support brain function, and vitamin D, which is important for bone health and may also play a role in nerve function, is particularly important for Parkinson's patients.

Calcium-rich foods like dairy products and leafy greens support bone density and muscle contraction, contributing to overall mobility and balance.

Finally, B vitamins, particularly B6 and B12, are crucial for nerve function and energy metabolism. Foods like whole grains, nuts, and fortified cereals provide these essential vitamins, supporting neurological health and energy levels in Parkinson's patients. Minerals like iron and calcium are vital for muscle function and bone strength. Iron-rich foods like lean red meat and spinach can help combat fatigue, a common symptom of Parkinson's.

THE USE OF SUPPLEMENTS TO HELP WITH SYMPTOM MANAGEMENT

In addition to a patient's diet, supplements can help with specific symptoms or fill in nutrient gaps. For example, coenzyme Q10, an antioxidant that supports cellular energy production and may help slow down the progression of Parkinson's symptoms, omega-3 supplements derived from flaxseed or fish oil, offer anti-inflammatory benefits that can support joint health and cognitive function, and vitamin D supplements are often advised to maintain immune system function and bone strength, especially for those with limited sun exposure.

Whey protein, in particular, is easily absorbed and used by the body to support muscle repair and growth; however, it's important to consult with a healthcare provider before starting any new supplement regimen to ensure compatibility with existing medications and individual health needs. Supplements should always be used as part of a comprehensive treatment plan that includes a balanced diet and regular exercise. Parkinson's patients who struggle to maintain muscle mass due to decreased appetite or swallowing difficulties may need to take protein supplements.

TECHNIQUES FOR COOKING THAT MAINTAIN NUTRIENTS

Cooking techniques have a big impact on food's nutritional value, especially for people with Parkinson's disease who need to consume as many nutrients as possible. For example, steaming vegetables helps to retain water-soluble vitamins like vitamins C and B vitamins, which are important for energy metabolism and nerve function. Similarly, stir-frying vegetables quickly over high heat helps to retain the crunch and nutrients in vegetables like broccoli and bell peppers, which are important for digestive health because they provide antioxidants and fiber.

Poaching fish in broth or water helps retain omega-3 fatty acids without adding extra fat, promoting heart health and cognitive function. Slow-cooking stews or soups can break down tough fibers in vegetables and meats, making them easier to digest while maintaining nutrient density. Overall, choosing cooking methods that preserve nutrients ensures Parkinson's patients receive maximum nutritional benefits from their meals. Grilling or broiling lean meats like chicken or fish allows fat to drip away, reducing calorie intake while preserving protein and essential amino acids necessary for muscle health and energy maintenance.

RECIPES PACKED WITH VITAL MINERALS AND VITAMINS

Formulating vitamin and mineral-rich recipes can help people with Parkinson's disease eat a balanced diet and enjoy tasty meals. For example, a vitamin C and antioxidant-rich spinach and berry smoothie boosts immune system function and cellular repair, while a protein, fiber, and healthy fat combination in quinoa salad with avocado and chickpeas promotes satiety and digestive health.

These recipes, which taste great and guarantee that Parkinson's patients get the nutrients they need to manage their symptoms and maintain overall health, include baked sweet potatoes topped with Greek yogurt and walnuts, which provide vitamin A, calcium, and protein, supporting bone health and cognitive function; salmon with roasted vegetables, which provides omega-3 fatty acids, vitamin D, and minerals like potassium and magnesium, which support heart health and muscle function; and a fruit and yogurt parfait with granola.

INCLUDING PROTEIN FOR HEALTHY MUSCLES AND ENERGY

Lean protein sources like chicken, fish, and tofu contribute to muscle growth and repair; an omelet with spinach and feta cheese for breakfast offers a high-protein start to the day along with vital vitamins and minerals for general health. Protein is crucial for maintaining muscle health and providing sustained energy for Parkinson's patients, who may experience muscle stiffness and fatigue.

Protein-rich foods at every meal help Parkinson's patients manage symptoms like muscle weakness and fatigue while supporting optimal physical function and quality of life. Snacks like Greek yogurt with almonds or cottage cheese with fruit offer a quick and easy way to boost protein intake between meals, supporting muscle recovery and maintaining energy levels. Lunch or dinner should be grilled chicken or fish with quinoa and steamed vegetables for a balanced meal rich in protein, fiber, and nutrients essential for overall well-being.

CHAPTER FIVE

SIMPLE COOKING METHODS FOR PARKINSON'S DISEASE PATIENTS

Meal preparation can be made more manageable for those with Parkinson's disease by using simple and effective techniques. To start, arrange your workspace to reduce movement and confusion. Use utensils with ergonomic handles that are comfortable to grip, like large-handled knives and peelers. Choose recipes with minimal steps and use less-dexterity cooking methods like stir-frying or one-pot meals. Dividing tasks into smaller, manageable steps can also help you stay focused and feel less exhausted.

Efficient cooking methods include pre-chopping ingredients or using pre-cut vegetables; using pots and pans with two handles for better stability and ease of movement; using non-stick cookware or lining baking trays with parchment paper to reduce sticking and cleanup; and using longer-handled utensils or investing in automatic stirring devices for recipes that call for stirring to lessen physical strain.

EQUIPMENT & TOOLS FOR PREPARING MEALS

For people with Parkinson's disease, meal preparation can be made much easier with the right tools and equipment. Start with ergonomic kitchen tools like electric can openers, jar openers, and easy-grip measuring cups; these tools minimize wrist and hand strain by reducing the need to grip and twist. You can also buy food processors or blenders to quickly chop and puree ingredients.

To enhance control and stability when cooking, think about utilizing adapted kitchen tools like larger-handled or weighted utensils. Appliances that make cooking easier, like slow cookers or instant pots, allow for longer cooking times without constant attention. When it comes to chopping, think about using non-slip cutting boards or stabilizing mats to prevent accidents and encourage safety in the kitchen.

Parkinson's patients can benefit from meal preparation in advance by planning their meals for the week and preparing ingredients in bulk, such as chopping and washing vegetables or portioning ingredients for recipes. Precooked meals or ingredients can be stored in freezer-friendly containers for convenient reheating or assembly on busy days. Label containers with reheating instructions.

Make use of batch cooking techniques by increasing the number of your favorite recipes and freezing individual servings for easy meals. This method helps you avoid having to cook and clean up after meals every day, which makes mealtimes less stressful.

You can also reduce waste and maximize efficiency by planning meals that use leftovers to create new dishes. By preparing ahead of time, you can enjoy healthy meals without the hassle of cooking every day.

HOW TO ADJUST RECIPES TO FIT SPECIFIC DIETARY REQUIREMENTS

The key to managing Parkinson's disease is to modify recipes to suit specific dietary needs. Begin by determining dietary preferences or restrictions and choosing recipes that fit these needs.

Replace ingredients to accommodate allergies or intolerances, like dairy-free alternatives or gluten-free flour. Modify seasoning and spices to improve flavor without sacrificing dietary restrictions.

Change portion sizes to control calorie intake and maintain a balanced diet. Add more fruits, vegetables, and whole grains to recipes to boost nutritional value. Use herbs and spices instead of salt to enhance taste and reduce sodium intake, which is beneficial for overall health management. Experiment with different cooking methods, such as steaming or grilling, to reduce fat content or increase nutrient retention in meals.

When cooking for Parkinson's patients, fatigue management is essential. Start by planning cooking sessions for when the patient's energy is at its peak, which is usually in the morning or after a period of rest. Take short breaks in between tasks to avoid burnout and keep concentration. Set priorities and assign easier tasks to family members or caregivers to reduce workload.

Make the most of your kitchen's layout by placing frequently used items in convenient locations to reduce strain and movement; use anti-fatigue mats or comfortable seating options to ease standing discomfort; drink plenty of water and eat wholesome snacks like fruits or nuts to stay energized while preparing meals; and think about utilizing accessible tools like rolling stools or adjustable countertops to make your workspace more accessible.

Cooking for Parkinson's disease can be made more manageable and pleasurable by putting these useful strategies and advice into practice.

Make sure to simplify tasks, make use of the appropriate tools, and plan to maximize efficiency and minimize physical strain. Modify recipes to suit specific dietary requirements and effectively handle fatigue to support general well-being and meal enjoyment.

CHAPTER SIX

ORGANIZING LUNCHES FOR PARTICULAR EVENTS

Planning and being prepared arc essential when following a Parkinson's disease diet; start by choosing recipes that emphasize foods high in nutrients and low in fats, sugars, and sodium; add a range of vibrant fruits and vegetables, lean proteins, whole grains, and healthy fats to create a well-balanced meal that promotes general health and wellbeing.

Make it easier by making a meal plan that consists of Parkinson's diet-recommended appetizers, main courses, side dishes, and desserts. Cooking techniques like baking, grilling, or steaming cut down on saturated fat intake. Take into account food texture because people with Parkinson's disease may find softer foods easier to chew and swallow. Include family and friends in meal planning to make sure everyone's tastes and dietary requirements are met.

Last but not least, plan as much as you can to reduce stress on the day of the celebration. Create a list of the ingredients, cooking tools, and serving utensils required for each recipe. If at all possible, assign tasks to guests so that everyone can participate in the celebration while the meal preparation is fun and easy.

RECIPES FOR FAMILY GET-TOGETHERS

Celebrate with Parkinson's disease-friendly meals at holiday get-togethers. Opt for recipes that highlight seasonal flavors and ingredients while still adhering to dietary guidelines. For appetizers, try healthy and quick-to-prepare fresh vegetable platters with hummus or yogurt-based dips. To add some variation, serve whole grain crackers or bread alongside.

Plan lean meats like chicken or turkey for main courses, and include plant-based proteins like beans or lentils in soups or stews. Play around with herbs and spices to add flavor without adding too much salt or fat. Roasted veggies or salads with homemade dressings make great side dishes and are high in nutrients.

Desserts can include fruit salads, yogurt parfaits with berries and nuts, or baked fruit crisps with oats and a tiny bit of natural sweetener. These options not only satiate sweet tooths but also fit into a well-balanced meal plan. Watch portion sizes to prevent overindulging, and urge guests to take their time and enjoy the flavors and textures of each dish.

ADAPTING CLASSIC RECIPES TO MEET DIETARY REQUIREMENTS

Creative cooking and a thorough understanding of nutritional needs are necessary when modifying classic recipes to meet Parkinson's dietary needs. To begin, identify key ingredients that can be substituted or adjusted to lower fat, sodium, and sugar content. For instance, you can season dishes with spices or low-sodium broth instead of salt. Try baking or grilling alternative cooking methods to achieve similar flavors without sacrificing nutritional value.

For creamy dishes, use Greek yogurt or pureed vegetables instead of heavy cream to maintain texture while reducing saturated fats. Add plenty of vegetables to dishes for added vitamins, minerals, and antioxidants. Replace ingredients to incorporate more fiber-rich options, such as whole grains or legumes, into recipes traditionally high in refined carbohydrates.

Test recipes to make sure the adapted foods are tasty and filling. Get input from loved ones and friends to improve the recipes even more. Record the successful adjustments for future use. Build a customized cookbook of Parkinson 's-friendly recipes that you can eat for special occasions and regular meals.

IDEAS FOR ENJOYING THE HOLIDAYS WITH FRIENDS AND FAMILY

Thanksgiving is a happy occasion that can be made inclusive and pleasurable while adhering to a Parkinson's disease diet. Arrange social events, like games, storytelling, or music sessions that emphasize social interaction over food consumption. Select locations that can accommodate dietary requirements, or host get-togethers at home where meal preparation can be managed.

Set a festive table with decorations that go with the celebration's theme to create a warm and inviting atmosphere. Offer flavored water, herbal teas, and fresh fruit juices as healthy beverage options instead of sugary drinks or alcohol. Serve delicious and nutritious Parkinson's disease-friendly meal options to guests so they feel included and satisfied.

Invite guests to help prepare meals or bring dietary-compliant dishes to create a cooperative and encouraging atmosphere. Discuss the significance of the occasion and stress the value of staying healthy while spending time with loved ones.

STRATEGIES FOR HANDLING DIETARY LIMITATIONS DURING HOLIDAYS

Planning and communicating are essential to making sure that everyone's dietary needs are satisfied during celebrations.

Begin by alerting hosts or guests to any special dietary needs associated with Parkinson's disease, such as a preference for low-sodium, low-sugar, and nutrient-dense foods. Offer to bring dishes that comply with these guidelines to make sure there are plenty of options available.

To assist guests in making educated decisions about what they eat, compile a list of ingredients used in recipes; clearly label dishes to indicate what's in them, especially if there are any allergies or special dietary requirements; or organize a buffet-style meal where guests can choose items based on their dietary requirements and preferences.

Talk openly about dietary restrictions to build empathy and support among guests. Offer substitute ingredients or cooking techniques that can satisfy different dietary needs without sacrificing nutritional value.

CHAPTER SEVEN

MEAL PLANNING: BREAKFASTS RECIPES

HEALTHY BREAKFAST CHOICES TO BEGIN THE DAY

Boost your energy levels and support overall health by starting your day with a variety of nutrient-dense breakfast options that will fuel your body and mind. A balanced breakfast should include whole grains, fruits, and lean proteins. Whole grain options, such as oatmeal or whole wheat toast, provide fiber for sustained energy, while fruits, like berries or bananas, offer essential vitamins and antioxidants. Lean protein sources, like eggs, Greek yogurt, or tofu, help you feel full and satisfied until your next meal. Finally, stay hydrated with water or herbal tea to boost metabolism and aid in digestion.

Try different combinations to make your breakfasts enticing and fun. For a fuss-free, on-the-go breakfast, try overnight oats with chia seeds and almond milk. Smoothies with spinach, avocado, and protein powder are another excellent choice for a nutrient-dense, quick meal. If you're in the mood for something warm and savory, try preparing a vegetable omelet with mushrooms, spinach, and a sprinkle of cheese. If you're craving something sweet, try whole grain pancakes or waffles with fresh fruit on top and a drizzle of honey or maple syrup.

SIMPLE AND FAST BREAKFAST RECIPES

Keeping simple and quick breakfast recipes on hand guarantees that you can still enjoy a satisfying meal without the hassle. Overnight oats are an absolute game changer; just combine oats, milk (or dairy-free alternative), and your preferred toppings (nuts, seeds, and fruit) in a jar the night before, then grab and go for a satisfying and tasty breakfast the next morning. Smoothie bowls are another quick option; blend frozen fruits, spinach or kale, Greek yogurt or almond milk, and a scoop of protein powder for a cool start to the day. Garnish with granola, nuts, and seeds for extra crunch and flavor.

Meal prep is easy with egg muffins: beat eggs with veggies like bell peppers, onions, and spinach; pour into muffin tins and bake until set; store in the refrigerator or freezer for a quick, high-protein breakfast you can reheat in a matter of minutes; avocado toast is a stylish, yet straightforward option: mash ripe avocado on whole grain toast, sprinkle with salt, pepper, and olive oil; top with a poached or fried egg for additional flavor and protein; these recipes are not only time-saving, but they also supply the necessary nutrients to power your morning routine.

WORTH OF A WELL-BALANCED BREAKFAST

Skipping breakfast can result in lethargy, poor concentration, and overeating later in the day. A balanced breakfast sets the tone for the day by providing essential nutrients and energy to support optimal physical and mental performance. A variety of food groups should be included to ensure you receive a range of vitamins, minerals, and macronutrients necessary for overall health.

Fiber from whole grains like oats and whole wheat aids in digestion and helps you feel fuller for longer. Vitamins, antioxidants, and hydration from fruits and vegetables are essential for the immune system and cell repair.

Healthy fats from sources like avocados, nuts, and seeds support brain health and mood regulation. Balancing carbohydrates, proteins, and fats in your breakfast promotes steady energy levels throughout the morning. Whether you prefer sweet or savory options, aim to include a mix of nutrient-dense foods to optimize your breakfast routine. Protein-rich foods like eggs, Greek yogurt, and nuts stabilize blood sugar levels and prevent cravings for unhealthy snacks.

RECIPES FOR INCREASED VITALITY

Make the most of your energy levels by consuming these nutrient-dense breakfast recipes that will fuel your body for the day. Smoothies are an excellent way to include a range of ingredients that offer sustained energy.

For a cool and revitalizing smoothie, blend spinach, banana, berries, almond milk, and a scoop of protein powder. For a heartier option, try a breakfast quinoa bowl, which is made by cooking quinoa in almond milk and then topping it with nuts, seeds, dried fruit, and honey.

A substantial amount of protein and essential nutrients can be found in egg-based dishes like veggie-packed frittata or scrambled eggs with vegetables. To enhance flavor and nutritional value, add bell peppers, tomatoes, and leafy greens. Chia seed pudding made with almond milk and topped with fresh fruit and nuts is another great option for a breakfast that satisfies cravings and releases energy gradually.

BREAKFAST CONCEPTS FIT FOR A RANGE OF DIETARY RESTRICTIONS

It's now easier than ever to find breakfast ideas that satisfy a variety of dietary requirements. For example, people on a gluten-free diet can replace traditional oats in recipes like overnight oats or granola with gluten-free oats; for avocado toast or breakfast sandwiches, use gluten-free bread; and smoothie bowls packed with fruits, vegetables, and seeds that are naturally gluten-free and vegan-friendly can be made with dairy-free milk alternatives like almond or coconut milk.

If you're vegetarian or vegan, you can use plant-based protein sources like tofu, tempeh, and legumes in recipes like tofu scrambles or breakfast burritos. Nut butters and seeds add protein and healthy fats to smoothies, oatmeal, or toast. If you're lactose intolerant, you can use lactose-free yogurt or milk substitutes like soy, almond, or oat milk in recipes without losing flavor or nutrition. Try experimenting with different combinations of ingredients to make breakfast options that will satisfy your palate and nutritional requirements.

CHOOSING HEALTHFUL LUNCH AND DINNER OPTIONS

Parkinson's patients should prioritize nutrient-dense foods that support overall health and effectively manage symptoms when choosing lunch and dinner options. Antioxidants, vitamins, and minerals are important for supporting brain health and minimizing oxidative stress, and a balanced plate usually consists of lean proteins like fish or poultry, whole grains like quinoa or brown rice for sustained energy, and an abundance of colorful vegetables for fiber and vital nutrients.

Easier meal prep is achieved by batch-cooking basic ingredients, such as roasted vegetables or grilled chicken breast, which can be used in a variety of recipes during the week. Baking, grilling, or steaming are good ways to preserve nutrients without adding too much fat, and adding healthy fats from nuts, avocados, or olive oil can help with brain function and general health.

To support optimal health and symptom management for Parkinson's patients, a typical healthy dinner might be grilled salmon with quinoa and roasted vegetables. This meal provides omega-3 fatty acids from the salmon, protein, and fiber from the quinoa, and a variety of vitamins and minerals from the vegetables. It's important to customize portion sizes to individual needs and preferences while focusing on whole, minimally processed foods.

ONE-POT DINNERS FOR EASE

Parkinson's patients and their caregivers can benefit from one-pot meals, which are simple, convenient, and nutritious meals that can be made in just one pot or pan, minimizing cleanup and cooking time. One-pot meals that are appropriate for Parkinson's patients include soups, stews, and casseroles that can be tailored with nutrient-dense ingredients to meet dietary needs.

For example, to make a hearty vegetable stew, sauté onions and garlic in olive oil, then add diced carrots, potatoes, and bell peppers.

Add lean protein (diced chicken or beans) for extra nutrition, and simmer with low-sodium broth and flavorings like herbs. Whole grains (like barley or quinoa) can also be added to one-pot meals for extra fiber and long-lasting energy.

Caretakers can provide patients with nourishing, easily digestible, and enjoyable meals by combining a variety of colorful vegetables, lean proteins, and whole grains into one-pot recipes.

These meals not only make meal planning easier but also guarantee a well-balanced diet that supports overall health and effectively manages Parkinson's symptoms.

DINNER RECIPES THAT ARE FAMILY-FRIENDLY

Incorporating familiar flavors and textures while focusing on nutrient-dense ingredients ensures that meals are both satisfying and supportive of overall health. Family-friendly dinners can include dishes like grilled chicken with mixed greens and whole-grain pasta, which provide a balance of protein, fiber, and essential vitamins. Creating dinners that satisfy the tastes of loved ones and the nutritional needs of Parkinson's patients can be accomplished with thoughtful recipe choices.

For example, to make nutritious spaghetti bolognese, brown lean ground beef or turkey with onions and garlic, then add tomato sauce and simmer with diced vegetables, such as carrots and mushrooms, to enhance flavor and nutrition. For a lighter version that still satisfies hunger and provides essential nutrients, serve over zucchini noodles or whole-grain spaghetti.

Incorporating family members into meal preparation and taking into account their preferences allows caregivers to establish a supportive environment that promotes healthy eating habits for all members of the family. This strategy not only makes mealtimes more enjoyable but also builds a sense of support and connection within the family, which benefits Parkinson's patients and their loved ones' general well-being.

Parkinson's patients should make quick lunches that are nutrient-dense, satisfying, and easy to make to maintain their energy levels throughout the day. Choosing nutrient-dense, simple foods such as salads, wraps, or sandwiches can supply essential nutrients without requiring a lot of preparation time. Lean proteins, whole grains, and an abundance of vegetables guarantee well-balanced meals that support satiety and general well-being.

A quick and healthy lunch option is to make a spinach and grilled chicken salad with quinoa and colorful veggies. Toss spinach with cooked quinoa, diced grilled chicken, cucumbers, cherry tomatoes, and a little olive oil and lemon juice for flavor. This salad is packed with protein, fiber, vitamins, and minerals and is very simple to put together.

Another easy lunch option is a whole grain wrap stuffed with hummus, thinly sliced carrots and bell peppers, mixed greens, and sliced chicken or turkey.

Whole grain wraps are adaptable and can be tailored with preferred ingredients to meet personal preferences while maintaining a well-rounded nutritional profile.

HEALTHY MEALS TO CONTROL SYMPTOMS ALL DAY LONG

To ensure adequate nutrition and symptom management, meals should include a combination of lean proteins, complex carbohydrates, healthy fats, and a variety of vegetables. Balancing meals can help stabilize energy levels and minimize fluctuations in mood and cognition. Meals should be balanced to provide sustained energy and support overall health for Parkinson's patients.

Make oatmeal with Greek yogurt, fresh berries, and a sprinkling of nuts or seeds for breakfast. This combination of protein-rich yogurt, antioxidant-rich berries, and fiber-rich oats supports brain health and increases satiety. Nuts and seeds also provide healthy fats that aid in the absorption of nutrients and contribute to overall well-being.

To sustain energy levels and reduce appetite in between meals, try including snacks such as fresh fruit with nut butter, yogurt with granola, or vegetable sticks with hummus. These snacks are full of vital nutrients and can help Parkinson's patients avoid overindulging during main meals, which promotes healthy weight management and overall well-being.

Caregivers can help Parkinson's patients manage their symptoms and maintain optimal health by emphasizing balanced meals that include a variety of nutrient-dense foods. Meals can be customized to meet dietary needs and individual preferences, ensuring that each meal promotes overall well-being and improves the quality of life for both patients and their caregivers.

HEALTHY SNACK IDEAS TO REDUCE CRAVINGS

For those with Parkinson's disease, finding nourishing snack options that not only satiate cravings but also support overall health can be crucial. These snacks should ideally be balanced in terms of nutrients, offering sustained energy without resulting in blood sugar spikes. A great option is a handful of mixed nuts, like almonds, walnuts, and pistachios, which are rich in antioxidants, healthy fats, and protein. These nuts can be combined with a piece of fruit, like an apple or banana, to add extra fiber and natural sweetness, supporting digestive health. Greek yogurt topped with berries and honey is another excellent option, combining protein, probiotics, and antioxidants in a tasty and satisfying treat.

To satisfy a savory craving, try homemade hummus with raw vegetable sticks, such as carrots, celery, and bell peppers. The hummus adds fiber and protein, and the veggies provide vitamins and minerals that are important for overall health. Whole grain crackers with avocado spread and a sprinkling of sunflower seeds can also be a crunchy, nutrient-dense snack that promotes heart health and satiety. These snack ideas not only effectively satisfy cravings but also support a balanced Parkinson's diet by guaranteeing consistent energy levels and meeting nutritional needs all day long.

DESSERTS THAT ARE HEALTHFUL BUT NOT GUILTY

A simple fruit salad with a variety of berries and a sprinkle of cinnamon can be a refreshing and guilt-free dessert option. Another idea is a homemade yogurt parfait with layers of Greek yogurt, fresh fruits, and a small amount of granola for added crunch and fiber. Desserts for people with Parkinson's disease should be delicious and health-conscious. Berries, for example, are rich in antioxidants and low in natural sugars, so choosing desserts that incorporate them can satisfy a sweet tooth while providing beneficial nutrients.

If you're in the mood for something a little more decadent, dark chocolate-covered strawberry is a rich and healthy option. Dark chocolate has antioxidants and may be good for heart health, and strawberries are high in fiber and vitamin C. Baked apples packed with a blend of oats, nuts, and a little honey or maple syrup make for a filling dessert that's also high in complex carbohydrates and healthy fats that support overall wellbeing. People with Parkinson's disease can enjoy desserts without sacrificing their dietary objectives by selecting desserts that emphasize whole, natural ingredients with minimal added sugars.

THE VALUE OF PORTION MANAGEMENT IN SNACKS

For people with Parkinson's disease, maintaining appropriate portion control is essential because it helps control calories consumed and weight, both of which can affect general health. When snacking, it's critical to pay attention to serving sizes to prevent calorie overconsumption and possible blood sugar swings. One useful tactic is to portion snacks into smaller containers or bags in advance so that each serving is suitable and ready to go when hunger strikes.

A portion-controlled serving of whole grain crackers with a small amount of cheese or nut butter offers a satisfying blend of nutrients without excess calories; similarly, pre-cut portions of vegetables with hummus or guacamole ensure a balanced snack that supports nutritional goals while promoting satiety. By practicing portion control with snacks, people with Parkinson's can effectively manage their dietary intake, support overall health, and enhance their quality of life. Thus, incorporating balanced snacks that combine protein, healthy fats, and carbohydrates in moderation can help maintain steady energy levels throughout the day.

RECIPES FOR DESSERTS AND SNACKS MADE AT HOME

Making homemade snacks and desserts gives people with Parkinson's disease complete control over the ingredients, so they can match dietary requirements and preferences. For example, homemade granola bars are a simple and adaptable recipe that can be customized with oats, nuts, seeds, and dried fruits. These bars are easy to make in large quantities and offer a convenient, high-fiber, high-fat snack option. Another idea is homemade trail mix, which combines roasted nuts, seeds, and a small quantity of dark chocolate chips for a filling and high-nutrient snack.

If you have a sweet tooth, you can make healthier oatmeal cookies by baking them with whole-grain flour, oats, and natural sweeteners like honey or mashed bananas. You can make these cookies in smaller portions to help with portion control and still satisfy your sweet tooth. You can also make a rich and silky chocolate banana ice cream by blending frozen bananas with cocoa powder and a little almond milk. This is a low-sugar, naturally sweetened dessert that tastes great. Parkinson's patients can prioritize their diets by trying out these tasty recipes for snacks and desserts.

LIMITING SUGAR CONSUMPTION WHILE INDULGING IN SWEETS

To support overall health and effectively manage symptoms, people with Parkinson's disease must control their sugar intake.

One way to do this is to limit added sugars in the diet by choosing desserts and snacks that are naturally sweetened with fruits or small amounts of natural sweeteners. For example, choosing fresh fruit salads or fruit smoothies made with unsweetened almond milk and a handful of spinach provides natural sweetness from fruits without additional sugar.

Sweets made at home can be made with less sugar overall by replacing refined sugar with options like stevia, honey, or maple syrup. Desserts like chia seed pudding, which is made with unsweetened almond milk and a dash of vanilla extract, are rich, creamy, and naturally low in sugar and high in fiber. Desserts can also benefit from the flavor boost that comes from adding cinnamon or nutmeg, which tastes great without adding extra sugar and helps achieve dietary goals.

Parkinson's disease patients can improve their quality of life, support overall health, and maintain better control over their diets by reducing their intake of sugar and choosing naturally sweetened snacks and desserts.

DRINKS THAT ARE HYDRATING FOR PEOPLE WITH PARKINSON'S

To support bodily functions and maintain fluid balance, people with Parkinson's disease need to stay hydrated. One practical strategy is to incorporate hydrating drinks into daily routines. For example, plain water infused with citrus slices or mint for a refreshing twist is a hydrating option for Parkinson's patients. Herbal teas, such as chamomile or ginger tea, not only hydrate but also have soothing properties that can help alleviate digestive discomfort or nausea, which are common issues for Parkinson's patients.

For those who prefer a little taste, diluted fruit juices can be a hydrating option when consumed in moderation and as long as they are low in added sugars. Including these hydrating drinks throughout the day helps maintain optimal hydration levels, supporting overall well-being and possibly alleviating some

Parkinson's symptoms related to dehydration. Another great option is coconut water because it naturally contains electrolytes.

Smoothies are an easy and nutrient-dense way for people with Parkinson's disease to get more of the nutrients they need while still enjoying tasty flavors. A simple but effective smoothie can be made with spinach, banana, almond milk, and a scoop of protein powder. This combination gives you fiber, potassium, and protein—all of which are necessary for healthy muscles and general energy levels. A handful of berries increases the amount of antioxidants in the smoothie, which may help reduce oxidative stress related to Parkinson's disease.

Nut butter smoothies with ingredients like almond butter, banana, oats, and milk offer a balanced blend of protein, healthy fats, and complex carbohydrates, supporting sustained energy throughout the day. These nutrient-packed smoothies can be enjoyed as a meal replacement or a satisfying snack, promoting overall health and well-being for Parkinson's patients. For variation, a tropical smoothie with pineapple, mango, coconut water, and Greek yogurt offers a refreshing taste while providing hydration, vitamins, and probiotics for gut health.

THE VALUE OF MAINTAINING HYDRATION DURING THE DAY

Maintaining proper hydration is critical for people with Parkinson's disease to support overall health and effectively manage symptoms. Dehydration can exacerbate muscle stiffness and fatigue, common challenges for those living with Parkinson's. Therefore, stressing the importance of drinking water and hydrating beverages throughout the day is crucial. Proper hydration helps regulate body temperature, lubricate joints, and aid in digestion, essential functions that can be affected by Parkinson's symptoms.

Parkinson's patients can support their overall health and potentially alleviate some symptoms associated with dehydration by prioritizing hydration throughout the day. Other strategies to encourage regular hydration include setting reminders to drink fluids, keeping a water bottle nearby for easy access, and incorporating hydrating snacks like fruits with high water content. Urine color can also serve as a simple indicator of hydration status; pale yellow urine suggests adequate hydration, while dark yellow urine may indicate dehydration.

SUGGESTIONS FOR WARM AND CHILLED DRINKS

Cold beverages like iced herbal teas, homemade fruit smoothies, and infused water with cucumber or berries offer refreshing alternatives during warmer weather or when thirst strikes. A variety of hot and cold beverages gives Parkinson's patients options to suit their preferences and needs throughout the day. Hot options like herbal teas, bone broth, or warm milk with honey not only hydrate but also offer comfort and relaxation, which can be beneficial for managing stress and promoting restful sleep.

Incorporating a variety of hot and cold beverages into daily routines helps Parkinson's patients stay hydrated while enjoying a variety of flavors and textures to support overall well-being.

Those with Parkinson's disease can benefit from a wide variety of beverages as long as they maintain their nutritional intake and hydration levels. One way to do this is by experimenting with different temperature preferences and flavor combinations.

DRINKS TO LIMIT OR STEER CLEAR OFF TO MANAGE SYMPTOMS

While staying hydrated is important, patients with Parkinson's disease should be aware of some drinks that can make their condition worse or interfere with their medications. Caffeine-containing drinks, like coffee or energy drinks, can make tremors worse and disrupt sleep, which can affect how well symptoms are managed overall. Alcohol should also be avoided or consumed in moderation as it can interact with

Parkinson's medications and make balance and coordination problems worse.

Water, herbal teas, or diluted fruit juices ensure hydration without the negative effects associated with sugary or caffeinated beverages; making informed beverage choices can support symptom management and overall health for people living with Parkinson's disease. Sugary drinks like soda or sweetened juices should also be limited because they have the potential to spike blood sugar levels and contribute to weight gain, which can impact mobility and overall health.

CHAPTER EIGHT

THE BENEFITS OF EXERCISE FOR MANAGING PARKINSON'S SYMPTOMS

Frequent exercise helps manage the symptoms of Parkinson's disease by improving mobility, balance, and overall quality of life. Strength training exercises like weightlifting or resistance bands can improve muscle strength and flexibility, reducing the risk of falls and improving daily activities. Flexibility exercises like yoga or stretching can help maintain the range of motion in joints and muscles, which can become stiff due to Parkinson's. Aerobic exercises like walking, cycling, or swimming help maintain cardiovascular health and enhance endurance.

Exercise not only helps manage physical symptoms but also fosters neuroplasticity, the brain's capacity to adapt and form new connections. Including a variety of exercises into a weekly routine is beneficial, with an emphasis on aerobic, strength, and flexibility training. One should speak with a healthcare provider or a physical therapist to customize an exercise program that suits individual needs and abilities. Lastly, regular physical activity is safe and effective in managing Parkinson's disease symptoms.

SLEEP IS ESSENTIAL FOR GENERAL HEALTH

A regular sleep schedule and the creation of a sleep-friendly environment can help improve sleep quality. Quality sleep is essential for overall health, especially for people with Parkinson's disease, as it contributes to physical, mental, and emotional well-being. Sleep helps regulate neurotransmitters, including dopamine, which is crucial in managing Parkinson's symptoms. Adequate sleep supports cognitive function, memory consolidation, and mood regulation, all of which can be affected by Parkinson's disease.

Parkinson's patients' sleep patterns can be disrupted by a variety of factors, including side effects from medications, motor symptoms like tremors or stiffness, and sleep disorders like insomnia or sleep apnea. These factors can be managed through medication adjustments, relaxation techniques, and lifestyle modifications, all of which can help patients sleep better. Good sleep hygiene, which includes minimizing caffeine and alcohol intake, setting up a comfortable sleeping environment, and adhering to a regular sleep schedule, can also improve sleep quality and support the overall health of people with Parkinson's disease.

CONTROLLING STRESS AND HOW IT AFFECTS SYMPTOMS

For people with Parkinson's disease, stress management is essential because stress aggravates motor symptoms and negatively impacts general well-being. Deep breathing exercises, mindfulness, and meditation are some techniques that help lower stress levels and encourage relaxation. Exercises like yoga or tai chi also help lower stress levels and improve mood by releasing endorphins, which are the body's natural stress relievers. Hobbies, social activities, and time spent in nature can also help lower stress levels.

To effectively manage stress, people with Parkinson's disease must recognize their triggers and create coping mechanisms to deal with them. Support groups and counseling can offer important emotional support as well as helpful coping strategies. People with Parkinson's disease who prioritize self-care and maintain a balanced lifestyle that includes enough sleep, food, and social support can also improve their overall quality of life.

COMMON QUESTIONS REGARDING PARKINSON'S DISEASE AND DIET

A balanced diet rich in fruits, vegetables, whole grains, and lean proteins can provide essential nutrients and support overall health; foods high in antioxidants, like berries, leafy greens, and nuts, may help protect against oxidative stress, which is thought to contribute to the progression of Parkinson's disease; maintaining a consistent eating schedule and staying hydrated are important for supporting the effectiveness of medication and digestive health.

A registered dietitian can provide personalized nutrition guidance and address specific dietary concerns or nutritional deficiencies. It's also important to monitor medication interactions with certain foods or supplements and make adjustments as recommended by a healthcare provider. People with Parkinson's disease can support overall health and well-being by prioritizing nutrition and making informed dietary choices. Some people with the disease may have difficulty chewing or swallowing, so it's important to modify food textures or consider liquid supplements as needed.

SOURCES OF ADDITIONAL INFORMATION AND SUPPORT

For people with Parkinson's disease and their caregivers, it is critical to have access to trustworthy resources and support networks. The Parkinson's Foundation, the Michael J. Fox Foundation, and neighborhood Parkinson's support groups are some of the organizations that provide invaluable information, educational materials, and social support. Online forums and social media groups can link people with

Parkinson's disease to others going through similar struggles, offering emotional support and useful guidance.

Participating in clinical trials or research studies may also offer opportunities to access cutting-edge treatments and contribute to the advancement of Parkinson's disease research. Understanding the most recent advancements in Parkinson's research and treatment options empowers people with Parkinson's disease to make informed decisions about their health and well-being. Healthcare providers, including neurologists, movement disorder specialists, and physical therapists, play a crucial role in managing Parkinson's disease and can provide personalized guidance and treatment options.